The Complete Air Fryer Recipe Book

Boost Your Metabolism and Enjoy Your Meals with Incredibly Tasty Air Fryer Dishes

Kira Hamm

TABLE OF CONTENT

this book has been derived from various sources. Please consult a licensed professional before attempting any techniques outlined in this book.

By reading this document, the reader agrees that under no circumstances is the author responsible for any losses, direct or indirect, which are incurred as a result of the use of information contained within this document, including, but not limited to, — errors, omissions, or inaccuracies.

Turkey Chili

Preparation Time:15 minutes

Cooking Time: 30 minutes

Serves 6

Ingredients:

- 1 tablespoon extra-virgin olive oil
- 1 pound (454 g) lean ground turkey
- 1 large onion, diced
- 3 garlic cloves, minced
- 1 red bell pepper, seeded and diced
- 1 cup chopped celery
- 2 tablespoons chili powder
- 1 tablespoon ground cumin
- 1 (28-ounce / 794-g) can reduced-salt diced tomatoes
- 1 (15-ounce / 425-g) can low-sodium kidney beans, drained and rinsed
- 2 cups low-sodium chicken broth

Directions:

1. In a large pot, heat the oil over medium heat. Add the turkey, onion, and garlic, and cook, stirring regularly, until the turkey is cooked through.

2. Add the bell pepper, celery, chili powder, and cumin. Stir well and continue to cook for 1 minute.
3. Add the tomatoes with their liquid, kidney beans, and chicken broth. Bring to a boil, reduce the heat to low, and simmer for 20 minutes.

Nutrition: calories: 276 | fat: 10g | protein: 23g | carbs: 27g | sugars: 7g | fiber: 8g | sodium: 556mg

Turkey Divan Casserole

Preparation Time: 10 minutes

Cooking Time: 50 minutes

Serves 6

Ingredients:

- Nonstick cooking spray
- 3 teaspoons extra-virgin olive oil, divided
- 1 pound (454 g) turkey cutlets
- ¼ teaspoon freshly ground black pepper, divided
- ¼ cup chopped onion
- 2 garlic cloves, minced
- 2 tablespoons whole-wheat flour
- 1 cup unsweetened plain almond milk
- 1 cup low-sodium chicken broth
- ½ cup shredded Swiss cheese, divided
- ½ teaspoon dried thyme
- 4 cups chopped broccoli
- ¼ cup coarsely ground almonds

Directions:

1. In a skillet, heat 1 teaspoon of oil over medium heat. Season the turkey with the salt and 1/8 teaspoon of pepper. Sauté the

turkey cutlets for 5 to 7 minutes on each side until cooked through. Transfer to a cutting board, cool briefly, and cut into bite-size pieces.

2. In the same pan, heat the remaining 2 teaspoons of oil over medium-high heat. Sauté the onion for 3 minutes until it begins to soften. Add the garlic and continue cooking for another minute.

3. Stir in the flour and mix well. Whisk in the almond milk, broth, and remaining 1/8 teaspoon of pepper, and continue whisking until smooth. Add ¼ cup of cheese and the thyme, and continue stirring until the cheese is melted.

4. In the baking dish, arrange the broccoli on the bottom. Cover with half the sauce. Place the turkey pieces on top of the broccoli, and cover with the remaining sauce. Sprinkle with the remaining ¼ cup of cheese and the ground almonds.

5. Bake for 35 minutes until the sauce is bubbly and the top is browned.

Nutrition: calories: 207 | fat: 8g | protein: 25g |

carbs: 9g | sugars: 2g | fiber: 3g | sodium: 128mg

Turkey Broccoli Casserole

Preparation Time:10 Minutes

Cooking Time: 30 minutes

Servings: 6

Ingredients:

- 2-1/2 cups turkey breast, cubed and cooked
- 16 oz. broccoli, chopped and drained
- 1-1/2 cups of milk, fat-free
- 1 cup cheddar cheese, low-fat, shredded
- 10 oz. cream of chicken soup. low sodium and low fat
- What you will need from the store cupboard:
- 8 oz. egg substitute
- ¼ teaspoon of poultry seasoning
- ¼ cup of sour cream, low fat
- 2 cups of seasoned stuffing cubes

Directions:

1. Bring together the egg substitute, soup, milk, pepper, sour cream, salt, and poultry seasoning in a big bowl.

2. Now stir in the broccoli, turkey, ¾ cup of cheese and stuffing cubes.
3. Transfer to a baking dish. Apply cooking spray.
4. Bake for 10 minutes. Sprinkle the remaining cheese.
5. Bake for another 5 minutes.
6. Keep it aside for 5 minutes. Serve.

Nutrition: Calories 303, Carbohydrates 26g, Fiber 3g, Sugar 0.8g, Cholesterol 72mg, Total Fat 7g, Protein 33g

Homemade Turkey Breakfast Sausage

Preparation Time: 10 minutes

Cooking Time: 10 minutes

Serving: 8

Ingredients:

- 1-pound lean ground turkey
- ½ teaspoon dried sage
- ½ teaspoon dried thyme
- ½ teaspoon freshly ground black pepper
- ¼ teaspoon ground fennel seeds
- 1 teaspoon extra-virgin olive oil

Directions:

1. In a large mixing bowl, combine the ground turkey, salt, sage, thyme, pepper, and fennel. Mix well.
2. Shape the meat into 8 small, round patties.
3. Heat the olive oil in a skillet over medium-high heat. Cook the patties in the skillet for 3 to 4 minutes on each side until browned and cooked through.

4. Serve warm, or store in an airtight container in the refrigerator for up to 3 days or in the freezer for up to 1 month.

Nutrition: Calories: 92; Total Fat: 5g; Protein: 11g; Carbohydrates: 0g; Sugars: 0g; Fiber: 0g; Sodium: 156mg

Sweet Potato, Onion, and Turkey Sausage Hash

Preparation Time:10 minutes

Cooking Time: 25 minutes

Serving: 4

Ingredients:

- 1 tablespoon extra-virgin oil
- 2 medium sweet potatoes, cut into ½-inch dice
- ½ recipe Homemade Turkey Breakfast Sausage (here)
- 1 small onion, chopped
- ½ red bell pepper, seeded and chopped
- 2 garlic cloves, minced

Directions:

1. In a large skillet, heat the oil over medium-high heat. Add the sweet potatoes and cook, stirring occasionally, for 12 to 15 minutes until they brown and begin to soften.
2. Add the turkey sausage in bulk, onion, bell pepper, and garlic. Cook for 5 to 6 minutes

until the turkey sausage is cooked through and the vegetables soften.

3. Garnish with parsley and serve warm.

Nutrition: Calories: 190; Total Fat: 9g; Protein: 12g; Carbohydrates: 16g; Sugars: 7g; Fiber: 3g; Sodium: 197mg

Easy Turkey Breakfast Patties

Preparation Time:10 minutes

Cooking Time: 10 minutes

Serves 8

Ingredients:

- 1 pound (454 g) lean ground turkey
- ½ teaspoon dried thyme
- ½ teaspoon dried sage
- ½ teaspoon salt
- ½ teaspoon freshly ground black pepper
- ¼ teaspoon ground fennel seeds
- 1 teaspoon extra-virgin olive oil

Directions:

1. Mix the ground turkey, thyme, sage, salt, pepper, and fennel in a large bowl, and stir until well combined.
2. Form the turkey mixture into 8 equal-sized patties with your hands.
3. In a skillet, heat the olive oil over medium-high heat. Cook the patties for 3 to 4 minutes per side until cooked through.

Nutrition: Calories: 91 | fat: 4.8g | protein: 11.2g |

carbs: 0.1g | fiber: 0.1g | sugar: 0g| sodium: 155mg

Turkey Spinach Patties

Preparation Time:10 minutes

Cooking Time: 20 minutes

Servings:4

Ingredients:

- 1 lb. ground turkey
- 1 1/2 cups fresh spinach, chopped
- 1 tsp Italian seasoning
- 1 tbsp olive oil
- 1 tbsp garlic, minced
- 4 oz feta cheese, crumbled

Directions:

1. Add ground turkey and remaining Ingredients into the mixing bowl and mix until well combined.
2. Make four equal shapes of patties from turkey mixture and place it into the air fryer basket.
3. Cook turkey patties for 20 minutes.

Nutritional: Calories 336 Fat 22.4 g Carbohydrates 2.4 g Sugar 1.3 g Protein 35.5 g Cholesterol 142 mg

Tasty Turkey Fajitas

Preparation Time:10 minutes

Cooking Time: 20 minutes

Servings:4

Ingredients:

- 1 lb. turkey breast, boneless, skinless, and cut into 1/2-inch slices
- 1/4 cup fresh cilantro, chopped
- 1 jalapeno pepper, chopped
- 1 onion, sliced
- 2 bell pepper, sliced into strips
- 1 1/2 tbsp olive oil
- 2 lime juice
- 1/2 tsp onion powder
- 1 tsp garlic powder
- 1/2 tbsp oregano
- 1/2 tsp paprika
- 1 tbsp chili powder

Directions:

1. In a small bowl, mix together onion powder, garlic powder, oregano, paprika, cumin, chili powder, and pepper.

2. Squeeze one lime juice over turkey breast then sprinkle spice mixture over turkey breast.
3. Brush turkey breast with 1 tbsp olive oil and set aside.
4. Add onion and bell peppers into the medium bowl and toss with remaining oil.
5. Preheat the cosori air fryer to 375 F.
6. Add onion and bell peppers into the air fryer basket and cook for 8 minutes. Shake basket and cook for 5 minutes more.
7. Add jalapenos and cook for 5 minutes. Shake basket and add sliced turkey over vegetables and cook for 8 minutes.

Nutrition: Calories 211 Fat 7.8 g Carbohydrates 16.2 g Sugar 9.1 g Protein 20.9 g Cholesterol 49 mg

Turkey Broccoli Fritters

Preparation Time:10 minutes

Cooking Time: 10 minutes

Servings:8

Ingredients:

- 1 lb. turkey thighs, boneless, skinless cut into small pieces
- 2 cups broccoli florets, steamed and chopped
- 1 cup cheddar cheese, shredded
- 1/2 cup almond flour
- 1/2 tsp garlic powder
- 2 eggs, lightly beaten

Directions:

1. Spray air fryer basket with cooking spray.
2. Add turkey and remaining Ingredients into the mixing bowl and mix until well combined.
3. Make small fritters from the chicken mixture and place it into the air fryer basket.

4. Cook turkey fritters at 400 F for 8 minutes. Turn chicken fritters and cook for 2 minutes more.

Nutrition: Calories 199 Fat 10.9 g Carbohydrates 2.3 g Sugar 0.6 g Protein 22.4 g Cholesterol 106 mg

Spicy Turkey Wings

Preparation Time:10 minutes

Cooking Time: 30 minutes

Servings:4

Ingredients:

- 2 lbs. turkey wings
- 2 tsp garlic powder
- 4 tsp chili powder
- 3 tbsp olive oil

Directions:

1. Add turkey wings and remaining Ingredients into the zip-lock bag and shake well to coat.
2. Place turkey wings into the air fryer basket and cook at 380 F for 30 minutes. Toss chicken wings every 5 minutes.

Nutrition: Calories 534 Fat 27.8 g Carbohydrates 2.5 g Sugar 0.5 g Protein 66.2 g Cholesterol 202 mg

Nutritious Turkey & Veggies

Preparation Time: 10 minutes

Cooking Time: 10 minutes

Servings: 4

Ingredients:

- 1 lb. turkey breast, boneless & cut into bite-size pieces
- 1 tbsp Italian seasoning
- 1/2 tsp garlic powder
- 1/2 tsp chili powder
- 2 tbsp olive oil
- 2 garlic cloves, minced
- 1/2 onion, chopped
- 1 cup bell pepper, chopped
- 1 zucchini, chopped
- 1 cup broccoli florets

Directions:

1. Preheat the cosori air fryer to 400 F.
2. Add turkey and remaining Ingredients into the large mixing bowl and toss well.
3. Add turkey and veggies mixture into the air fryer basket and cook for 10 minutes or

until turkey is cooked. Shake air fryer basket halfway through.

Nutrition: Calories 235 Fat 11.2 g Carbohydrates 8 g Sugar 3.8 g Protein 25.9 g Cholesterol 75 mg

Turkey Spinach Meatballs

Preparation Time:10 minutes

Cooking Time: 10 minutes

Servings:4

Ingredients:

- 1 lb. ground turkey
- 3/4 cup almond flour
- 1/4 cup feta cheese, crumbled
- 2 tbsp parmesan cheese, grated
- 1/4 cup sun-dried tomatoes, drained
- 2 tsp garlic
- 3 cups baby spinach

Directions:

1. Add spinach, sun-dried tomatoes, and 1 tsp garlic into the food processor and process until a paste is formed.
2. Add spinach mixture into the large mixing bowl. Add remaining Ingredients into the bowl and mix until well combined.
3. Make small meatballs from mixture and place into the air fryer basket.
4. Cook meatballs at 400 F for 10 minutes.

Nutrition: Calories 303 Fat 14.7 g Carbohydrates 3.5

g Sugar 1 g Protein 38.4 g Cholesterol 114 mg

Tender Turkey Legs

Preparation Time: 10 minutes

Cooking Time: 27 minutes

Servings: 4

Ingredients:

- 4 turkey legs
- 1/4 tsp thyme
- 1/4 tsp oregano
- 1/4 tsp rosemary
- 1 tbsp butter

Directions:

1. Season turkey legs with pepper and salt.
2. In a small bowl, mix together butter, thyme, oregano, and rosemary.
3. Rub the butter mixture all over turkey legs.
4. Place turkey legs into the air fryer basket and cook for 27 minutes.

Nutrition: Calories 182 Fat 9.9 g Carbohydrates 1.9 g Sugar 0.1 g Protein 20.2 g Cholesterol 68 mg

Grilled Quail

Preparation Time 10 minutes

Cooking Time:1 hour 55 minutes

Serving: 6

Ingredients:

- 6 ounces of quail
- 1 cup of bouillon
- Bacon strips
- Stuffing
- Worcestershire sauce
- Pepper and salt

Directions:

1. Split the quail.
2. Sprinkle pepper and salt on the quail.
3. Add stuffing and bouillon
4. Wrap quail and bacon strip together.
5. Sprinkle with Worcestershire sauce.
6. Place it in the Power XL Air Fryer Grill basket.
7. Set the Power XL Air Fryer Grill to grill function.
8. Cook for 1 hour 45 minutes.

9. Serve immediately or allow cooling before serving.

Nutrition: Calories: 134kcal, Fat: 5g, Carb: 3g, Proteins: 21g

Turkey Breasts

Preparation Time: 5 minutes

Cooking Time: 1 hour

Servings: 4

Ingredients:

- Boneless turkey breast – 3 lbs.
- Mayonnaise – ¼ cup
- Poultry seasoning – 2 tsps.
- Salt and pepper to taste
- Garlic powder – 1/2 tsp.

Directions:

1. Preheat the air fryer to 360F. Season the turkey with mayonnaise, seasoning, salt, garlic powder, and black pepper. Cook the turkey in the air fryer for 1 hour at 360F.

2. Turning after every 15 minutes. The turkey is done when it reaches 165F.

Nutrition: Calories 558 Carbs 1g Fat 18g Protein 98g

BBQ Chicken Breasts

Preparation Time:5 minutes

Cooking Time: 15 minutes

Servings: 4

Ingredients:

- Boneless, skinless chicken breast – 4, about 6 oz. each
- BBQ seasoning – 2 tbsps.
- Cooking spray

Directions:

1. Rub the chicken with BBQ seasoning and marinate in the refrigerator for 45 minutes. Preheat the air fryer at 400F. Grease the basket with oil and place the chicken.
2. Then spray oil on top. Cook for 13 to 14 minutes. Flipping at the halfway mark. Serve.

Nutrition: Calories 131 Carbs 2g Fat 3g Protein 24g

Rotisserie Chicken

Preparation Time: 5 minutes

Cooking Time: 1 hour

Servings: 4

Ingredients:

- Whole chicken – 1, cleaned and patted dry
- Olive oil – 2 tbsps.
- Seasoned salt – 1 tbsp.

Directions:

1. Remove the giblet packet from the cavity. Rub the chicken with oil and salt. Place in the air fryer basket, breast-side down. Cook at 350F for 30 minutes.
2. Then flip and cook another 30 minutes. Chicken is done when it reaches 165F.

Nutrition: Calories 534 Carbs 0g Fat 36g Protein 35g

Honey-Mustard Chicken Breasts

Preparation Time: 5 minutes

Cooking Time: 25 minutes

Servings: 6

Ingredients:

- Boneless, skinless chicken breasts – 6 (6-oz, each)
- Fresh rosemary – 2 tbsps. minced
- Honey – 3 tbsps.
- Dijon mustard – 1 tbsp.
- Salt and pepper to taste

Directions:

1. Combine the mustard, honey, pepper, rosemary and salt in a bowl. Rub the chicken with this mixture.
2. Grease the air fryer basket with oil. Air fry the chicken at 350F for 20 to 24 minutes or until the chicken reaches 165F. Serve.

Nutrition: Calories 236 Carbs 9.8g Fat 5g Protein 38g

Chicken Parmesan Wings

Preparation Time: 5 minutes

Cooking Time: 15 minutes

Servings: 4

Ingredients:

- Chicken wings – 2 lbs. cut into drumettes, pat dried
- Parmesan – 1/2 cup, plus 6 tbsps. grated
- Herbs de Provence – 1 tsp.
- Paprika – 1 tsp.
- Salt to taste

Directions:

1. Combine the parmesan, herbs, paprika, and salt in a bowl and rub the chicken with this mixture. Preheat the air fryer at 350F.
2. Grease the basket with cooking spray. Cook for 15 minutes. Flip once at the halfway mark. Garnish with parmesan and serve.

Nutrition: Calories 490 Carbs 1g Fat 22g Protein 72g

Air Fryer Chicken

Preparation Time: 5 minutes

Cooking Time: 30 minutes

Servings: 4

Ingredients:

- Chicken wings – 2 lbs.
- Salt and pepper to taste
- Cooking spray

Directions:

1. Flavor the chicken wings with salt and pepper. Grease the air fryer basket with cooking spray. Add chicken wings and cook at 400F for 35 minutes.
2. Flip 3 Times during cooking for even cooking. Serve.

Nutrition: Calories 277 Carbs 1g Fat 8g Protein 50g

Whole Chicken

Preparation Time: 5 minutes

Cooking Time: 40 minutes

Servings: 6

Ingredients:

- Whole chicken – 1 (2 1/2 pounds) washed and pat dried
- Dry rub – 2 tbsps.
- Salt – 1 tsp.
- Cooking spray

Directions:

1. Preheat the air fryer at 350F. Rub the dry rub on the chicken. Then rub with salt. Cook it at 350°F for 45 minutes. After 30 minutes, flip the chicken and finish cooking.
2. Chicken is done when it reaches 165F.

Nutrition: Calories 412 Carbs 1g Fat 28g Protein 35g

Honey Duck Breasts

Preparation Time: 5 minutes

Cooking Time: 25 minutes

Servings: 2

Ingredients:

- Smoked duck breast – 1, halved
- Honey – 1 tsp.
- Tomato paste – 1 tsp.
- Mustard – 1 tbsp.
- Apple vinegar – 1/2 tsp.

Directions:

1. Mix tomato paste, honey, mustard, and vinegar in a bowl. Whisk well. Add duck breast pieces and coat well. Cook in the air fryer at 370F for 15 minutes.
2. Remove the duck breast from the air fryer and add to the honey mixture. Coat again. Cook again at 370F for 6 minutes. Serve.

Nutrition: Calories 274 Carbs 22g Fat 11g Protein 13g

Creamy Coconut Chicken

Preparation Time: 5 minutes

Cooking Time: 20 minutes

Servings: 4

Ingredients:

- Big chicken legs – 4
- Turmeric powder – 5 tsps.
- Ginger – 2 tbsps. grated
- Salt and black pepper to taste
- Coconut cream – 4 tbsps.

Directions:

1. In a bowl, mix salt, pepper, ginger, turmeric, and cream. Whisk. Add chicken pieces, coat and marinate for 2 hours.
2. Transfer chicken to the preheated air fryer and cook at 370F for 25 minutes. Serve.

Nutrition: Calories 300 Carbs 22g Fat 4g Protein 20g

Buffalo Chicken Tenders

Preparation Time:5 minutes

Cooking Time: 20 minutes

Servings: 4

Ingredients:

- Boneless, skinless chicken tenders – 1 pound - Hot sauce – ¼ cup
- Pork rinds – 1 1/2 ounces, finely ground - Chili powder – 1 tsp.
- Garlic powder – 1 tsp.

Directions:

1. Put the chicken breasts in a bowl and pour hot sauce over them. Toss to coat. Mix ground pork rinds, chili powder and garlic powder in another bowl.
2. Place each tender in the ground pork rinds, and coat well. With wet hands, press down the pork rinds into the chicken. Place the tender in a single layer into the air fryer basket. Cook at 375F for 20 minutes. Flip once. Serve.

Nutrition: Calories 160 Carbs 0.6g Fat 4.4g Protein 27.3g

Teriyaki Wings

Preparation Time: 5 minutes

Cooking Time: 20 minutes

Servings: 4

Ingredients:

- Chicken wings – 2 pounds
- Teriyaki sauce – 1/2 cup
- Minced garlic – 2 tsp.
- Ground ginger - ¼ tsp.
- Baking powder – 2 tsp.

Directions:

1. Except for the baking powder, place all ingredients in a bowl and marinate for 1 hour in the refrigerator. Place wings into the air fryer basket and sprinkle with baking powder.
2. Gently rub into wings. Cook at 400F for 25 minutes. Shake the basket two- or three- Times during cooking. Serve.

Nutrition: Calories 446 Carbs 3.1g Fat 29.8g Protein 41.8g

Lemony Drumsticks

Preparation Time: 5 minutes

Cooking Time: 20 minutes

Servings: 2

Ingredients:

- Baking powder – 2 tsps.
- Garlic powder – 1/2 tsp.
- Chicken drumsticks – 8
- Salted butter – 4 tbsps. melted
- Lemon pepper seasoning – 1 tbsp.

Directions:

1. Sprinkle garlic powder and baking powder over drumsticks and rub into chicken skin. Place drumsticks into the air fryer basket. Cook at 375F for 25 minutes. Flip the drumsticks once halfway through the Cooking Time.
2. Remove when cooked. Mix seasoning and butter in a bowl. Add drumsticks to the bowl and toss to coat. Serve.

Nutrition: Calories 532 Carbs 1.2g Fat 32.3g Protein 48.3g

Parmesan Chicken Tenders

Preparation Time:5 minutes

Cooking Time: 10 minutes

Servings: 4

Ingredients:

- 1 pound chicken tenderloins
- 3 large egg whites
- 1/2 cup Italian-style bread crumbs
- ¼ cup grated Parmesan cheese

Directions:

1. Preparing the ingredients. Spray the Cuisinart air fryer basket with olive oil. Trim off any white fat from the chicken tenders. In a bowl, whisk the egg whites until frothy. In a separate small mixing bowl, combine the bread crumbs and Parmesan cheese. Mix well.

2. Dip the chicken tenders into the egg mixture, then into the Parmesan and bread crumbs. Shake off any excess breading. Place the chicken tenders in the greased Cuisinart air fryer basket in a single layer.

Generously spray the chicken with olive oil to avoid powdery, uncooked breading.

3. Air Frying. Set the temperature of your Cuisinart AF to 370°F. Set the Timer and bake for 4 minutes. Using tongs, flip the chicken tenders and bake for 4 minutes more. Check that the chicken has reached an internal temperature of 165°F. Add Cooking Time if needed. Once the chicken is fully cooked, plate, serve, and enjoy.

Nutrition: Calories: 210 Fat: 4g Saturated fat: 1g Carbohydrate: 10g Fiber: 1g Sugar: 1g Protein: 33g

Easy Lemon Chicken Thighs

Preparation Time: 5 minutes

Cooking Time: 10 minutes

Servings: 4

Ingredients:

- Salt and black pepper to taste
- 2 tablespoons olive oil
- 2 tablespoons Italian seasoning
- 2 tablespoons freshly squeezed lemon juice
- 1 lemon, sliced

Directions:

1. Place the chicken thighs in a medium mixing bowl and season them with the salt and pepper. Add the olive oil, Italian seasoning, and lemon juice and toss until the chicken thighs are thoroughly coated with oil. Add the sliced lemons. Place the chicken thighs into the air fryer basket in a single layer.

2. Set the temperature of your AF to 350°F. Set the Timer and cook for 10 minutes. Using tongs, flip the chicken. Reset the

Timer and cook for 10 minutes more. Check that the chicken has reached an internal temperature of 165°F. Add Cooking Time if needed. Once the chicken is fully cooked, plate, serve, and enjoy.

Nutrition: Calories 325 Carbs 1g Fat 26g Protein 20g

Air Fryer Grilled Chicken Breasts

Preparation Time: 5 minutes

Cooking Time: 14 minutes

Servings: 4

Ingredients:

- 1/2 teaspoon garlic powder
- salt and black pepper to taste
- 1 teaspoon dried parsley
- 2 tablespoons olive oil, divided
- 3 boneless, skinless chicken breasts

Directions:

1. Preparing the ingredients. In a small bowl, combine together the garlic powder, salt, pepper, and parsley. Using 1 tablespoon of olive oil and half of the seasoning mix, rub each chicken breast with oil and seasonings. Place the chicken breast in the air fryer basket.

2. Air Frying. Set the temperature of your Cuisinart AF to 370°F. Set the Timer and grill for 7 minutes.

3. Using tongs, flip the chicken and brush the remaining olive oil and spices onto the chicken. Reset the Timer and grill for 7 minutes more. Check that the chicken has reached an internal temperature of 165°F. Add Cooking Time if needed.

4. When the chicken is cooked, transfer it to a platter and serve.

Nutrition: Calories 182 Carbs 0g Fat 9g Protein 26g

Perfect Chicken Parmesan

Preparation Time: 5 Minutes

Cooking Time: 25 Minutes

Servings: 2

Ingredients:

- 2 large white meat chicken breasts, approximately 5-6 ounces
- 1 cup of breadcrumbs (Panko brand works well)
- 2 medium-sized eggs
- Pinch of salt and pepper
- 1 tablespoon of dried oregano
- 1 cup of marinara sauce
- 2 slices of provolone cheese
- 1 tablespoon of parmesan cheese

Directions:

1. Preparing the ingredients. Cover the basket of the Power air fryer XL with a lining of tin foil, leaving the edges uncovered to allow air to circulate through the basket.
2. Preheat the air fryer to 350 degrees.

3. In a mixing bowl, whisk the eggs wait until fluffy and until the yolks and whites are fully combined, and set aside.

4. In a separate mixing bowl, combine the breadcrumbs, oregano, salt and pepper, and set aside.

5. One by one, dip the raw chicken breasts into the bowl with dry ingredients, coating both sides; then submerge into the bowl with wet ingredients, then dip again into the dry ingredients. This double coating will ensure an extra crisp-and-delicious air-fry!

6. Lay the coated chicken breasts on the foil covering the Power air fryer Basket, in a single flat layer.

7. Air Frying. Set the Power air fryer XL Timer for 10 minutes.

8. After 10 minutes, the air fryer will turn off and the chicken should be mid-way cooked and the breaded coating starting to brown.

9. Use tongs, turn each piece of chicken over to ensure a full all-over fry.

10. Reset the air fryer to 320 degrees for another 10 minutes.

11. While the chicken is cooking, pour half the marinara sauce into a 7-inch heat-safe pan.

12. After 15 minutes, when the air fryer shuts off, remove the fried chicken breasts using tongs and set in the marinara-covered pan. Drizzle the remaining of the marinara sauce over the fried chicken, then place the slices of provolone cheese atop both of them and sprinkle the parmesan cheese over the entire pan.

13. Reset the air fryer to 350 degrees for 5 minutes.

14. After 5 minutes, when the air fryer shuts off, remove the dish from the air fryer using tongs or oven mitts. The chicken will be perfectly crisped and the cheese melted and lightly toasted. Serve while hot!

Nutrition: Calories: 210 Fat: 20g Protein: 18g Sugar: 0g

Honey and Wine Chicken Breasts

Preparation Time: 5 Minutes

Cooking Time: 15 Minutes

Servings: 4

Ingredients:

- 2 chicken breasts, rinsed and halved
- 1 tablespoon melted butter
- 1/2 teaspoon freshly ground pepper
- 3/4 teaspoon sea salt, or to taste
- 1 teaspoon paprika
- 1 teaspoon dried rosemary
- 2 tablespoons dry white wine
- 1 tablespoon honey

Directions:

1. Preparing the ingredients. Firstly, pat the chicken breasts dry. Lightly coat them with the melted butter.
2. Then, add the remaining ingredients.
3. Air Frying. Transfer them to the air fryer basket; bake about 15 minutes at 330 degrees F. Serve warm and enjoy

Nutrition: Calories: 189 Fat: 14g Protein: 11g Sugar:

Crispy Honey Garlic Chicken Wings

Preparation Time: 10 Minutes

Cooking Time: 25 Minutes

Servings: 8

Ingredients:

- 1/8 C. water
- 1/2 tsp. salt
- 4 tbsp. minced garlic
- ¼ C. vegan butter
- ¼ C. raw honey
- ¾ C. almond flour
- 16 chicken wings

Directions:

1. Preparing the ingredients. Rinse off and dry chicken wings well.
2. Spray air fryer basket with olive oil.
3. Coat chicken wings with almond flour and add coated wings to the Power air fryer XL.
4. Air Frying. Set temperature to 380°F, and set Time to 25 minutes. Cook shaking every 5 minutes.

5. When the Timer goes off, cook 5-10 minutes at 400 degrees till skin becomes crispy and dry.

6. As chicken cooks, melt butter in a saucepan and add garlic. Sauté garlic 5 minutes. Add salt and honey, simmering 20 minutes. Make sure to stir every so often, so the sauce does not burn. Add a bit of water after 15 minutes to ensure sauce does not harden.

7. Take out chicken wings from air fryer and coat in sauce. Enjoy!

Nutrition: Calories: 435 Fat: 19g Protein: 31g Sugar: 6g

Chicken-Fried Steak Supreme

Preparation Time: 10 Minutes

Cooking Time: 30 Minutes

Servings: 8

Ingredients:

- 1/2-pound chicken breast
- 1 cup of breadcrumbs (Panko brand works well)
- 2 medium-sized eggs
- Pinch of salt and pepper
- 1/2 tablespoon of ground thyme

Directions:

1. Preparing the ingredients. Cover the basket of the Power air fryer XL with a lining of tin foil, leaving the edges uncovered to allow air to circulate through the basket. Preheat the air fryer to 350 degrees. In a mixing bowl, beat the eggs until fluffy and until the yolks and whites are fully combined, and set aside. In a separate mixing bowl, combine the breadcrumbs, thyme, salt and pepper, and set aside. One by one, dip each

piece of raw steak into the bowl with dry ingredients, coating all sides; then submerge into the bowl with wet ingredients, then dip again into the dry ingredients. This double coating will ensure an extra crisp air fry. Lay the coated steak pieces on the foil covering the air-fryer basket, in a single flat layer.

2. Air Frying. Set the Power air fryer XL Timer for 15 minutes. After 15 minutes, the air fryer will turn off and the steak should be mid-way cooked and the breaded coating starting to brown. Using tongs, turn each piece of steak over to ensure a full all-over fry. Reset the air fryer to 320 degrees for 15 minutes. After 15 minutes, when the air fryer shuts off, remove the fried steak strips using tongs and set on a serving plate. Eat as soon as cool enough to handle and enjoy!

Nutrition: Calories: 180 Fat: 10g Protein: 15g Sugar: 0g

Lemon-Pepper Chicken Wings

Preparation Time: 10 Minutes

Cooking Time: 20 Minutes

Servings: 4

Ingredients:

- 8 whole chicken wings
- Juice of 1/2 lemon
- 1/2 teaspoon garlic powder
- 1 teaspoon onion powder
- Salt
- Pepper
- ¼ cup low-fat buttermilk
- 1/2 cup all-purpose flour
- Cooking oil

Directions:

1. Preparing the ingredients. Put the wings in a sealable plastic bag. Drizzle the wings with the lemon juice. Season the wings with the garlic powder, onion powder, and salt and pepper to taste.
2. Seal the bag. Shake thoroughly to combine the seasonings and coat the wings.

3. Pour the buttermilk and the flour into separate bowls large enough to dip the wings.

4. Spray the Power air fryer XL basket with cooking oil.

5. One at a Time, dip the wings in the buttermilk and then the flour.

6. Air Frying. Place the wings in the Power air fryer XL basket. It is okay to stack them on top of each other. Spray the wings with cooking oil, being sure to spray the bottom layer. Cook for 5 minutes.

7. Remove the basket and shake it to ensure all of the pieces will cook fully.

8. Return the basket to the Power air fryer XL and continue to cook the chicken. Repeat shaking every 5 minutes until a total of 20 minutes has passed.

9. Cool before serving.

Nutrition: Calories: 347 Fat: 12g Protein: 46g Fiber: 1g

Air Fried Chili Chicken

Preparation Time:25 minutes

Cooking Time: 10 minutes

Servings: 4

Ingredients:

- 1/2 tablespoon sesame oil
- 1 tablespoon low-sodium soy sauce
- 1 tablespoon cornstarch
- 450g chicken thighs, skinless, boneless, diced
- 1/2 tablespoon peanut oil
- 1 red onion, chopped
- 1 tablespoon minced fresh ginger
- 2 cups snow peas
- 1 tablespoon chili garlic sauce
- 1 mango, peeled, chopped
- 1/8 teaspoon sea salt
- 1/8 teaspoon black pepper

Directions:

1. In a large mixing bowl, combine sesame oil, soy sauce, cornstarch and chicken; let sit for at least 20 minutes.

2. In the pan from your air fryer toast oven, heat peanut oil and then sauté ginger and onion for about 2 minutes; add snow peas and stir fry for about 1 minute.

3. Add chicken with the marinade and transfer to your air fryer toast oven and air fry for 5 minutes at 350 degrees F or until chicken is browned.

4. Add chili sauce, mango and pepper and continue stir frying for 1 minute or until chicken is cooked through and mango is tender. Serve the stir fry over cooked brown rice.

Nutrition: Calories: 330 kcal, Carbs: 11.8 g, Fat: 24.1 g, Protein: 26 g.

Air Roasted Turkey

Preparation Time:10 minutes

Cooking Time: 40 minutes

Servings: 6

Ingredients:

- 2-3/4 pounds turkey breast
- 2 tablespoons unsalted butter
- 1 tablespoon chopped fresh rosemary
- 1 teaspoon chopped fresh chives
- 1 teaspoon minced fresh garlic
- 1/4 teaspoon black pepper
- 1/2 teaspoon salt

Directions:

1. Preheat your air fryer toast oven to 350 F.
2. In a bowl, mix together chives, rosemary, garlic, salt and pepper until well combined. Cut in butter and mash until well blended.
3. Rub the turkey breast with the herbed butter and then add to the air fryer toast oven basket; air roast for 20 minutes.
4. Turn the turkey breast and air roast for another 20 minutes.

5. Transfer the cooked turkey onto an aluminum foil and wrap; let rest for at least 10 minutes and then slice it up. Serve warm.

Nutrition: Calories: 263 kcal, Carbs: 0.3 g, Fat: 10.1 g, Protein: 40.2 g.

Air-Fried Lemon Chicken

Preparation Time:10 minutes

Cooking Time: 15 minutes

Servings: 4

Ingredients:

- 4 Boneless Skinless Chicken Breasts
- 1/2teaspoon organic cumin
- 1teaspoon sea salt (real salt)
- 1/4teaspoon black pepper
- 1/2cup butter, melted
- 1 lemons1/2 juiced, 1/2 thinly sliced
- 1cup chicken bone-broth
- 1can pitted green olives
- 1/2cup red onions, sliced

Directions:

1. Liberally season the chicken breasts with sea salt, cumin and black pepper
2. Preheat your air fryer toast oven to 370 degrees and brush the chicken breasts with the melted butter.
3. Air fry in the pan of your air fry toaster oven for about 5 minutes until evenly browned.

4. Add all remaining ingredients and air broil for 10 minutes.
5. Serve hot!

Nutrition: Calories: 310 kcal, Carbs: 10.2 g, Fat: 9.4 g, Protein: 21.8 g.

Baked Chicken Thighs

Preparation Time:15 minutes

Cooking Time: 35 minutes

Servings: 4

Ingredients:

- 500g chicken thighs
- 1 teaspoon red pepper flakes
- 1 teaspoon sweet paprika
- 1 teaspoon freshly ground black pepper
- 1 teaspoon dried oregano
- 1 teaspoon curry powder
- 1 tablespoon garlic powder
- 1-2 tablespoons coconut oil

Directions:

1. Start by preheating your air fryer toast oven to 370 degrees F and Preparing the basket of the fryer by lining it with parchment paper.
2. Combine all the spices in a small bowl then set aside.
3. Now arrange the thighs on your basket with the skin side down (remember to first pat the skin dry with kitchen towels).

4. Sprinkle the upper side of the chicken thighs with half the seasoning mix, flip them over and sprinkle the lower side with the remaining seasoning mix.

5. Bake for about 30 minutes until the chicken thighs are cooked through and the skin is crisp.

6. Turn once half way through Cooking Time:

7. To make the skin crispier, increase the heat to 400 degrees and bake for 5 more minutes.

8. Enjoy!

Nutrition: Calories: 281 kcal, Carbs: 3 g, Fat: 13 g, Protein: 36.8 g.

Turkey Wraps with Sauce

Preparation Time: 10 minutes

Cooking Time: 16 minutes

Servings: 6

Ingredients:

- Wraps
- 4 large collard leaves, stems removed
- 1 medium avocado, sliced
- 1/2 cucumber, thinly sliced
- 1 cup diced mango
- 6 large strawberries, thinly sliced
- 6 (200g) grilled turkey breasts, diced
- 24 mint leaves
- Dipping Sauce
- 2 tablespoons almond butter
- 2 tablespoons coconut cream
- 1 birds eye chili, finely chopped
- 2 tablespoons unsweetened applesauce
- 1/4 cup fresh lime juice
- 1 teaspoon sesame oil
- 1 tablespoon apple cider vinegar
- 1 tablespoon tahini
- 1 clove garlic, crushed

- 1 tablespoon grated fresh ginger
- 1/8 teaspoon sea salt

Directions:

1. For the chicken breasts:
2. Start by setting your air fryer toast oven to 350 degrees F.
3. Lightly coat the basket of the air fryer toast oven with oil.
4. Season the turkey with salt and pepper and arrange on the basket and air fry for 8 minutes on each side.
5. Once done, remove from air fryer toast oven and set on a platter to cool slightly then dice them up.
6. For the wraps:
7. Divide the veggies and diced turkey breasts equally among the four large collard leaves; fold bottom edges over the filling, and then both sides and roll very tightly up to the end of the leaves; secure with toothpicks and cut each in half.
8. Make the sauce:

9. Combine all the sauce ingredients in a blender and blend until very smooth. Divide between bowls and serve with the wraps.

Nutrition: Calories: 389 kcal, Carbs: 11.7 g, Fat: 38.2 g, Protein: 26 g.

Air Roasted Chicken Drumsticks

Preparation Time:10 minutes

Cooking Time: 20 minutes

Servings: 4

Ingredients:

- 1 tbsp. olive oil
- 1-1/2 red onions, diced
- 1-1/2 teaspoons salt
- 8 chicken drumsticks
- 1/2 teaspoon pepper
- 1/4 teaspoon chili powder
- 2 tablespoons thyme leaves
- Zest of 1/4 lemon
- 8 cloves of garlic
- 2/3 cup diced tinned tomatoes
- 2 tbsp. sweet balsamic vinegar

Directions:

1. Set your air fryer toast oven to 370 degrees F and add the oil, onions and 1/2 teaspoon of salt to the pan of your air fryer toast oven. Cook for 2 minutes until golden.

2. Add the chicken drumsticks and sprinkle with the rest of the salt, pepper and chili, then add the thyme, garlic cloves, and lemon zest; add in balsamic vinegar and tomatoes and spread the mixture between the drumsticks.
3. Air roast for about 20 minutes or until done to desire.
4. Serve the creamy chicken over rice, pasta or potatoes or with a side of vegetables.
5. Enjoy!

Nutrition: Calories: 329 kcal, Carbs: 13.3 g, Fat: 0.4 g, Protein: 20.8 g.

Scrumptious Turkey Wraps

Preparation Time:15 minutes

Cooking Time: 10 minutes

Servings: 4

Ingredients:

- 250g ground turkey
- 1/2 small onion, finely chopped
- 1 garlic clove, minced
- 2 tablespoons extra virgin olive oil
- 1 head lettuce
- 1 teaspoon cumin
- 1/2 tablespoon fresh ginger, sliced
- 2 tablespoons apple cider vinegar
- 2 tablespoons freshly chopped cilantro
- 1 teaspoon freshly ground black pepper
- 1 teaspoon sea salt

Directions:

1. Sauté garlic and onion in extra virgin olive oil until fragrant and translucent in your air fryer toast oven pan at 350 degrees F.
2. Add turkey and cook well for 5-8 minutes or until done to desire.

3. Add in the remaining ingredients and continue cooking for 5 minutes more.
4. To serve, ladle a spoonful of turkey mixture onto a lettuce leaf and wrap. Enjoy!

Nutrition: Calories: 197 kcal, Carbs: 8.4 g, Fat: 17.9 g, Protein: 13.4 g.

Air Roasted Whole Chicken

Preparation Time: 15 minutes

Cooking Time: 50 minutes

Servings: 12

Ingredients:

- 1 full chicken, dissected
- 2 tablespoons extra virgin olive oil
- 2 tablespoons chopped garlic
- 2 teaspoons sea salt
- 1 teaspoon pepper
- 1 tablespoon chopped fresh thyme
- 1 tablespoon chopped fresh rosemary
- Fruit Compote
- 1 apple, diced
- 1/2 cup red grapes, halved, seeds removed
- 12 dried apricots, sliced
- 16 dried figs, coarsely chopped
- 1/2 cup chopped red onion
- 1/2 cup cider vinegar
- 1/2 cup dry white wine
- 2 teaspoons liquid stevia
- 1/2 teaspoon salt

- 1/2 teaspoon pepper

Directions:

1. In a small bowl, stir together thyme, rosemary, garlic, salt and pepper and rub the mixture over the pork.

2. Light your air fryer toast oven and set it to 320°F, place the chicken on the basket and air roast for 10 minutes.

3. Increase the temperature and cook for another 10 minutes, turning the chicken pieces once. Increase the temperature one more Time to 400 degrees F and cook for 5 minutes to get a crispy finish.

4. Make Fruit Compote: In a saucepan, combine all ingredients and cook over medium heat, stirring, for about 25 minutes or until liquid is reduced to a quarter.

5. Once the chicken is cooked, serve hot with a ladle of fruit compote Enjoy!

Nutrition: Calories: 511 kcal, Carbs: 15 g, Fat: 36.8 g, Protein: 31.5

Grilled Catfish Fillets

Preparation Time: 10 minutes

Cooking Time:20 minutes

Servings: 5

Ingredients:

- 1 tbsp of parsley
- 5 fillets of catfish
- Sweet paprika
- 1 tbsp of olive oil
- Black pepper
- Salt
- 1 tbsp of lemon juice

Directions:

1. Drizzle catfish fillets with oil, pepper, salt, and paprika.
2. Place it in the Power XL Air Fryer Grill basket
3. Set the basket to position 6 in the Power XL Air Fryer Grill.
4. Set the Power XL Air Fryer Grill to Air fryer/Grill at 1450F.
5. Grill for about 20 minutes.
6. Serve immediately.

7. Serving Suggestions: Serve with lemon juice
8. Directions: & Cooking Tips: Rinse catfish fillet well

Nutrition: Calories: 320kcal, Fat: 10g, Carb: 0g, Proteins: 56g

Grilled Cod Fillets Mixed with Grapes Salad and Fennel

Preparation Time 10 minutes

Cooking Time:30 minutes

Servings: 3

Ingredients:

- 1 tbsp of olive oil
- 1/2 cup of pecans
- 1 sliced fennel bulb
- 3 black cod fillets
- Black pepper and salt
- 1 cup of grapes

Directions:

1. Rub oil all over the fish fillets.
2. Sprinkle with pepper and salt.
3. Place the fish on the Power XL Air Fryer Grill basket
4. Place the basket at position 6 in the Power XL Air Fryer Grill.
5. Set the Power XL Air Fryer Grill to Air fryer/Grill function at 1450F.

6. Grill for about 10 minutes

7. Mix grapes, pecans, oil, and fennel in another bowl, sprinkle with pepper and salt.

8. Place the mixture in the Power XL Air Fryer Grill basket.

9. Set the Power XL Air Fryer Grill to air fry function.

10.   Cook for about 5 minutes at 4000F.

11.   Serve cod with grape and fennel mix.

12.   Serving Suggestions: Serve with maple syrup

13.   Directions: & Cooking Tips: Divide the cod while serving

Nutrition: Calories: 154kcal, Fat: 3g, Carb: 0g, Proteins: 34g

Crispy Paprika Fish Fillets

Preparation Time:5 Minutes

Cooking Time: 15 Minutes

Servings: 4

Ingredients:

- 1/2 cup seasoned breadcrumbs
- 1 tablespoon balsamic vinegar
- 1/2 teaspoon seasoned salt
- 1 teaspoon paprika
- 1/2 teaspoon ground black pepper
- 1 teaspoon celery seed
- 2 fish fillets, halved
- 1 egg, beaten

Directions:

1. Preparing the ingredients. Pour the vinegar, salt, breadcrumbs, paprika, celery seeds and ground black pepper to your food processor. Leave it for 30 seconds.
2. Then cover the fish fillets using the beaten egg; then, put them into the breadcrumb's mixture.
3. Air Frying. Cook it at 350 degrees F for around 15 minutes.

Nutrition: Calories: 185; Fat: 11g; Protein: 21g; Sugar: 0g

Lemony Tuna

Preparation Time: 10 Minutes

Cooking Time: 10 Minutes

Servings: 4

Ingredients:

- 2 (6-ounce) cans water packed plain tuna
- 2 teaspoons Dijon mustard
- 1/2 cup breadcrumbs
- 1 tablespoon fresh lime juice
- 2 tablespoons fresh parsley, chopped
- 1 egg
- hot sauce
- 3 tablespoons canola oil
- Salt and freshly ground black pepper

Directions:

1. Preparing the ingredients. Get majority of the liquid from the canned tuna.
2. In a bowl, add the fish, mustard, crumbs, citrus juice, parsley, and hot sauce and mix till well combined. Add a little canola oil if it seems too dry. Add egg, salt and stir to combine. Make the patties from tuna

mixture. Refrigerate the tuna patties for about 2 hours.

3. Air Frying. Preheat the air fryer oven to 355 degrees F. Cook for about 10-12 minutes.

Nutrition: Calories: 345 Fat: 1g Protein: 18g Fiber: 4g

Grilled Soy Salmon Fillets

Preparation Time: 5 Minutes

Cooking Time: 8 Minutes

Servings: 4

Ingredients:

- 4 salmon fillets
- 1/4 teaspoon ground black pepper
- 1/2 teaspoon cayenne pepper
- 1/2 teaspoon salt
- 1 teaspoon onion powder
- 1 tablespoon fresh lemon juice
- 1/2 cup soy sauce
- 1/2 cup water
- 1 tablespoon honey
- 2 tablespoons extra-virgin olive oil

Directions:

1. Preparing the ingredients. Firstly, pat the salmon fillets dry using kitchen towels. Season the salmon with black pepper, cayenne pepper, salt, and onion powder.

2. To make the marinade, combine together the lemon juice, soy sauce, water, honey,

and olive oil. Marinate the salmon for at least 2 hours in your refrigerator.

3. Arrange the fish fillets on a grill basket in your XL air fryer oven.

4. Air Frying. Bake at 330 degrees for 8 to 9 minutes, or until salmon fillets are easily flaked with a fork.

5. Work with batches and serve warm.

Nutrition: Calories: 254 Fat: 4g Protein: 29g Fiber: 1g

Tender & Juicy Salmon

Preparation Time:10 minutes

Cooking Time: 7 minutes

Servings:2

Ingredients:

- 2 salmon fillets
- 2 tsp paprika
- 2 tsp olive oil
- Pepper
- Salt

Directions:

1. Rub salmon fillets with oil, paprika, pepper, and salt.
2. Place fillets into the air fryer basket and cook at 390 F for 7 minutes.
3. Serve and enjoy.

Nutrition: Calories 282 Fat 15.9 g Carbohydrates 1.2 g Sugar 0.2 g Protein 34.9 g Cholesterol 78 mg

Lemon Garlic White Fish

Preparation Time:10 minutes

Cooking Time: 10 minutes

Servings:2

Ingredients:

- 12 oz white fish fillets
- 1/2 tsp onion powder
- 1/2 tsp lemon pepper seasoning
- 1/2 tsp garlic powder
- Pepper
- Salt

Directions:

1. Preheat the cosori air fryer to 360 F.
2. Spray fish fillets with cooking spray and season with onion powder, lemon pepper seasoning, garlic powder, pepper, and salt.
3. Place parchment paper in the bottom of the air fryer basket. Place fish fillets into the air fryer basket and cook for 6-10 minutes.
4. Serve and enjoy.

Nutrition: Calories 298 Fat 12.8 g Carbohydrates 1.4 g Sugar 0.4 g Protein 41.9 g Cholesterol 131 mg

Parmesan White Fish Fillets

Preparation Time: 10 minutes

Cooking Time: 10 minutes

Servings: 4

Ingredients:

- 1 lb. white fish fillets
- 1/2 tsp lemon pepper seasoning
- 1/4 cup parmesan cheese
- 1/4 cup coconut flour

Directions:

1. In a shallow dish, mix together coconut flour, parmesan cheese, and lemon pepper seasoning.
2. Spray white fish fillets from both sides with cooking spray.
3. Coat fish fillets with coconut flour mixture.
4. Place coated fish fillets into the air fryer basket and cook at 400 F for 10 minutes. Turn fish fillets halfway through.
5. Serve and enjoy.

Nutrition: Calories 220 Fat 10 g Carbohydrates 0.9 g Sugar 0.1 g Protein 29.9 g Cholesterol 92 mg

Ginger Garlic Salmon

Preparation Time: 10 minutes

Cooking Time: 10 minutes

Servings: 2

Ingredients:

- 2 salmon fillets, boneless and skinless
- 2 tbsp mirin
- 2 tbsp soy sauce
- 1 tbsp olive oil
- 2 tbsp scallions, minced
- 1 tbsp ginger, grated
- 2 garlic cloves, minced

Directions:

1. Add salmon fillets into the zip-lock bag.
2. In a small bowl, mix together mirin, soy sauce, olive oil, scallions, ginger, and garlic and pour over salmon. Seal bag shake well and place it in the refrigerator for 30 minutes.
3. Place marinated salmon fillets into the air fryer basket and cook at 360 F for 10 minutes.
4. Serve and enjoy.

Nutrition: Calories 345 Fat 18.2 g Carbohydrates 11.6 g Sugar 4.5 g Protein 36.1 g Cholesterol 78 mg

Quick & Easy Salmon

Preparation Time: 10 minutes

Cooking Time: 12 minutes

Servings: 2

Ingredients:

- 2 salmon fillets
- 1/2 tsp hot sauce
- 3 tbsp coconut aminos
- 1 garlic clove, minced
- 1 tsp ginger, grated
- 1 tsp sesame seeds, toasted

Directions:

1. Add salmon fillets into the zip-lock bag.
2. Mix together hot sauce, coconut aminos, garlic, and ginger and pour over salmon. Seal bag and place in the refrigerator for 30 minutes.
3. Place marinated salmon fillets into the air fryer basket and cook at 400 F for 6 minutes.
4. Turn salmon and brush with marinade and cook for 6 minutes more or until cooked.
5. Serve and enjoy.

Nutrition: Calories 272 Fat 11.8 g Carbohydrates 6 g
Sugar 0.1 g Protein 35 g Cholesterol 78 mg

Healthy Salmon Patties

Preparation Time:10 minutes

Cooking Time: 7 minutes

Servings:2

Ingredients:

- 8 oz salmon fillet, minced
- 1/4 tsp garlic powder
- 1 egg, lightly beaten
- 1 lemon, sliced
- 1/8 tsp salt

Directions:

1. In a bowl, mix together mince salon, garlic powder, egg, and salt until well combined.
2. Make two patties from the salmon mixture.
3. Preheat the cosori air fryer to 390 F.
4. Place lemon sliced lemon on the bottom of the air fryer basket then place salmon patties on top.
5. Cook salmon patties for 7 minutes.
6. Serve and enjoy.

Nutrition: Calories 191 Fat 9.3 g Carbohydrates 3.1 g Sugar 1 g Protein 25.2 g Cholesterol 132 mg

Garlic Yogurt Salmon Fillets

Preparation Time:10 minutes

Cooking Time: 15 minutes

Servings:2

Ingredients:

- 2 salmon fillets
- 1/2 tsp garlic powder
- 1/4 cup Greek yogurt
- 1 tsp fresh lemon juice
- 1 tbsp fresh dill, chopped
- 1 lemon, sliced
- Pepper
- Salt

Directions:

1. Place lemon slices in the bottom of the air fryer basket.
2. Season salmon fillets with pepper and salt and place on a lemon slice in the air fryer basket.
3. Cook salmon fillets at 330 F for 15 minutes.
4. Place cooked salmon fillets on a serving plate.

5. Mix together yogurt, dill, lemon juice, and garlic powder.
6. Pour yogurt mixture overcooked salmon and serve.

Nutrition: Calories 277 Fat 11.9 g Carbohydrates 5.6 g Sugar 2.4 g Protein 38.8 g Cholesterol 80 mg

Parmesan Basil Salmon

Preparation Time: 10 minutes

Cooking Time: 7 minutes

Servings: 4

Ingredients:

- 4 salmon fillets
- 3 tbsp parmesan cheese, grated
- 5 fresh basil leaves, minced
- 3 tbsp mayonnaise
- 1/2 lemon juice
- Pepper
- Salt

Directions:

1. Preheat the cosori air fryer to 400 F.
2. Spray air fryer basket with cooking spray.
3. Season salmon with pepper, lemon juice, and salt.
4. In a small bowl, mix together chasse, basil, and mayonnaise.
5. Spread cheese mixture on top of salmon fillets. Place salmon fillets into the air fryer basket and cook for 7 minutes.
6. Serve and enjoy.

Nutrition: Calories 316 Fat 17.1 g Carbohydrates 3.2 g Sugar 0.8 g Protein 38.3 g Cholesterol 89 mg

Flavorful Curry Cod Fillets

Preparation Time:10 minutes

Cooking Time: 10 minutes

Servings:2

Ingredients:

- 2 cod fillets, defrosted and pat dry with a paper towel
- 1 tbsp Thai basil, sliced
- 1/8 tsp garlic powder
- 1/8 tsp paprika
- 1/4 tsp curry powder
- 1 tbsp butter, melted
- 1/8 tsp sea salt

Directions:

1. In a small bowl, mix together curry powder, garlic powder, paprika, and salt and set aside.
2. Line air fryer basket with aluminum foil.
3. Place cod fillets into the air fryer basket. Brush fillets with butter and sprinkles with dry spice mixture.

4. Cook at 360 F for 8 minutes. Drizzle with remaining butter and cook for 2 minutes more.

5. Garnish with basil and serve.

Nutrition: Calories 143 Fat 6.8 g Carbohydrates 0.4 g Sugar 0.1 g Protein 20.2 g Cholesterol 70 mg

Dukkah Crusted Salmon

Preparation Time:10 minutes

Cooking Time: 10 minutes

Servings:2

Ingredients:

- 1 tbsp dukkah
- 12 oz salmon fillets
- Pinch of salt

Directions:

1. Preheat the cosori air fryer to 390 F.
2. Season salmon with salt and sprinkle dukkah on top of salmon fillets.
3. Place salmon fillets into the air fryer basket and cook for 10 minutes.
4. Serve and enjoy.

Nutrition: Calories 248 Fat 12.3 g Carbohydrates 0.8 g Sugar 0 g Protein 33.8 g Cholesterol 75 mg

Herbed Salmon

Preparation Time:10 minutes

Cooking Time: 5 minutes

Servings:2

Ingredients:

- 8 oz salmon fillets
- 2 tbsp olive oil
- 1 tbsp lemon herb butter
- 1/4 tsp paprika
- 1 tsp Herb de Provence
- Pepper
- Salt

Directions:

1. In a small bowl, mix together paprika, Herb de Provence, pepper, and salt.
2. Rub salmon fillets with oil and spice mixture.
3. Place salmon fillets into the air fryer basket and cook at 390 F for 5-8 minutes.
4. Melt lemon herb butter and pour over salmon just before serving.

Nutrition: Calories 305 Fat 24.2 g Carbohydrates 1.2 g Sugar 0 g Protein 22.5 g Cholesterol 58 mg

Cod Steaks and Plum Sauce

Preparation time 10 minutes

Cooking Time:30 minutes

Servings: 3

Ingredients:

- 1 tbsp of plum sauce
- 1/2 tsp of garlic powder
- 3 large cod steaks
- Cooking spray
- 1/2 tsp of ginger powder
- Black pepper and salt
- 1/4 tsp of turmeric powder

Directions:

1. Drizzle the cod steaks with cooking spray.
2. Add pepper, ginger powder, salt, turmeric powder, and garlic powder.
3. Place the coated cod steaks in the Power XL Air Fryer Grill.
4. Set the function to Air fryer/Grill.
5. Grill for about 20 minutes at 3600F.
6. Flip while cooking for uniformity.
7. Heat plum sauce over medium heat for 2 minutes at reheat function.

8. Divide the cod steaks and serve immediately

9. Serving Suggestions: Serve with plum sauce

10. Directions: & Cooking Tips: Allow the coated shrimps to rest for some minutes before grilling.

Nutrition: Calories: 330kcal, Fat: 3g, Carb: 25g, Proteins: 30g

Flavored Grilled Salmon

Preparation Time 60 minutes

Cooking Time:8 minutes

Servings: 3

Ingredients:

- 3 chopped scallions
- 2 tbsp of lemon juice
- 1/3 cup of water
- 3 salmon fillets
- 1/2 tsp of garlic powder
- 2 tbsp of olive oil
- Black pepper and salt
- 1/3 cup of soy sauce
- 1/3 cup of brown sugar

Directions:

1. Mix soy sauce, sugar, lemon juice, salmon fillets in a bowl.
2. Add oil, garlic powder, pepper, water, and salt.
3. Put in the refrigerator for 1 hour
4. Place the salmon fillet in the Power XL Air Fryer Grill basket.

5. Set the Power XL Air Fryer Grill to Air fryer/Grill.

6. Allow to grill for about 8 minutes at 3600F.

Nutrition: Calories: 269kcal, Fat: 29g, Carb: 0g, Proteins: 51g

Grilled Lemony Saba Fish

Preparation Time 10 minutes

Cooking Time:8 minutes

Servings: 1

Ingredients:

- 2 tbsp of lemon juice
- 2 tbsp of minced garlic
- Black pepper and salt
- 2 tbsp of olive oil
- 4 saba fish fillet
- 3 chopped red chili pepper

Directions:

1. Drizzle the fish with oil, sprinkle salt and pepper.
2. Add chili, lemon juice, and garlic.
3. Toss well.
4. Place the fish on the Power XL Air Fryer Grill basket at position 6.
5. Set the Power XL Air Fryer Grill to Air fryer/Grill.
6. Grill for about 8 minutes at 3600F.
7. Flip while cooking
8. Serve immediately.

9. Serving Suggestions: Serve with fries and ketchup

10. Directions: & Cooking Tips: debone the fish fillet before adding Ingredients:

Nutrition: Calories: 231kcal, Fat: 17g, Carb: 0.2g, Proteins: 22g